The Sheld
Worry

G000065602

Dr Frank Tallis is an a
psychologist. He has held lecturing posts in clinical psychology and neuroscience at the Institute of Psychiatry, Psychology and Neuroscience (King's College, London), and is one of the country's leading authorities on obsessional states. He is the author of *Understanding Obsessions and Compulsions* (Sheldon Press, 1992) and *How to Stop Worrying* (Sheldon Press, reissued 2014), both of which are recommended on the Reading Well Books on Prescription scheme. He has written academic textbooks and over thirty academic papers, and is the author of several acclaimed novels.

Sheldon Short Guides

A full list of titles in the Overcoming Common Problems series is also available from Sheldon Press, 36 Causton Street, London SW1P 4ST and on our website at www.sheldonpress.co.uk

Depression
Dr Tim Cantopher

Memory Problems
Dr Sallie Baxendale

Phobias and Panic
Professor Kevin Gournay

Worry and Anxiety
Dr Frank Tallis

THE SHELDON SHORT GUIDE TO **WORRY** AND **ANXIETY**

Dr **Frank Tallis**

sheldon **PRESS**

First published in Great Britain in 2015

Sheldon Press
36 Causton Street
London SW1P 4ST
www.sheldonpress.co.uk

British Library Cataloguing-in-Publication Data
A catalogue record for this book is available from the
British Library

ISBN 978-1-84709-364-6
eBook ISBN 978-1-84709-365-3

Typeset by Fakenham Prepress Solutions, Fakenham,
Norfolk NR21 8NN
First printed in Great Britain by Ashford Colour Press
Subsequently digitally reprinted in Great Britain

eBook by Fakenham Prepress Solutions, Fakenham,
Norfolk NR21 8NN

Produced on paper from sustainable forests

Contents

1

What is worry?

What is worry? In spite of the fact that most people experience worry, professional mind-watchers like psychologists and psychiatrists have had very little to say about it. However, although professionals have failed to provide us with an agreed definition of worry, we can describe it and establish some common features of worry.

Two important features of worry are:

1 lack of control over repetitive bad thoughts;
2 a tendency to think things are going to get worse.

Jenny
Jenny couldn't concentrate. Her attention was constantly being interrupted by thoughts. Not just any thoughts, but bad, uncontrollable ones. The bad thoughts tended to get worse and worse, a process sometimes called 'catastrophizing'.

This book is about how you might learn to control your worries. We will not attempt to 'treat' or 'cure' worry, because this would be extremely unwise. As you are about to find out, in some situations worry might have very real advantages.

Does worry have a purpose?

Thoughts and feelings don't just happen. They occur for a reason.

Let's take a closer look at fear to illustrate this point. When you get frightened, certain things happen to your body. Chemicals, like adrenaline, are released into the blood, causing many changes: an increase in heart rate, 'heavy' breathing, sweating and the movement of blood away from some areas of the body – for example, the skin – to the muscles. These changes occur simply to prepare the body for action, and to equip us best for 'fight or flight'. An increased heart rate, and the movement of blood away from areas like the skin, will supply the muscles with all the chemicals required for vigorous activity – to fight 'harder' or run faster, depending on which response is chosen.

Fear, then, alters your body so that the chances of surviving a dangerous situation are improved. The idea that feelings have useful functions is not a new one. In fact Charles Darwin, the famous originator of the theory of evolution, was the first person to suggest that certain characteristics appear in both humans and animals because they have helped the species to survive. Clearly, fear is an extremely helpful emotion, albeit unpleasant.

Worry, then, is a response to a problem. Perhaps worry acts like an internal alarm system.

Another helpful effect of worry might be preparation. If thoughts and images relating to an unpleasant situation keep on coming into your mind, then this might help you to deal with the situation when it actually happens.

From the above we can see that worrying, although unpleasant, is in fact a perfectly normal thing to do. Worry might act as an alarm, telling you that a problem needs to be dealt with, while at the same time preparing you to deal with that problem. Worry is only a bad thing when it either starts unnecessarily or carries on for too long. Why, then, do some people worry more than others?

Why do I worry so much?

Everybody is different. We all have different beliefs and expectations. Because of these differences, no two people will react identically given the same situation.

Clearly, people who worry a lot tend to take a negative view of things and expect the worst. Why some people have this attribute and others don't is an extremely difficult question to answer. Perhaps it is a habit acquired during childhood. How we think and behave is strongly influenced by the way our parents think and behave. Parents provide children with example behaviours that tend to be copied. If we grow up in a family where it is normal to 'expect the worst', then it is quite likely that we will grow up expecting the worst too.

Although this sounds very plausible, note that at this stage we can only speculate on the influence of parenting on personality development and worry. Parental influence is probably just one of many factors that can shape our attitudes and beliefs. Others might include, for example, distressing life experiences. If you have had a lot of 'bad luck', and things keep on going wrong for you, then it will be difficult for you to maintain a positive picture of the world.

You can change this, using effective problem-solving techniques, which we'll look at next. Before we do so, let's remind ourselves how worry is triggered.

- A situation is thought to be threatening because it contains the possibility of one or more bad outcomes.
- Thoughts and images remind the individual that there is a problem that needs to be dealt with.
- If the individual fails to deal with the problem, worry will continue.
- But if the problem is dealt with, worry will stop. At worst, a few unpleasant thoughts might continue to be a nuisance before disappearing altogether.

Dealing with problems effectively

Situations that make us worry are problem situations. In a way, they should be treated like crossword puzzles or anagrams. If you're doing a puzzle of any kind, you have to think about it first. This process is known as **problem-solving**.

Everyday problem-solving can be broken down into a number of stages:

1 Define the problem. Be very specific: for example, 'I can't pay my heating bill.'
2 Think up as many ways of dealing with the problem as possible: for example, 'I could get a loan' or 'I could do some extra overtime at work.'
3 Decide which of these strategies is the best one.
4 Do it!

Worriers appear to be very good at defining problems but extremely bad at solving them. There are a number of reasons why this might be. However, research has shown that worriers tend to be slower than non-worriers when attempting to make a decision. This delay seems to stem from worriers' reluctance to make decisions unless they are absolutely sure that they are doing the right thing.

The longer it takes you to deal with a problem, the longer you will worry about it. Sometimes just deciding on a course of action will help you to stop worrying. If you make a decision to act in one way rather than another then you have reduced the uncertainty of your future.

In most situations, there just isn't enough evidence around to confirm that our decision is the best one. However, worriers are uncomfortable with this fact of life. Their decisions are delayed, because they go over things again and again in an attempt to be sure that what they are about to do is absolutely right. The relationship between problems, evidence requirements and worry is shown in Table 1.

Table 1 How unsolved problems keep worry going

The worrier becomes aware of a problem

↓

this
causes worry

↓

a decision is
needed to resolve the problem

↓

the worrier fails
to choose an appropriate plan

. . . because there's never enough evidence available
to guarantee that a particular plan is absolutely right

↓

the problem remains

↓

which leads to more worry

What do people worry about?

Research has shown that different worries can be divided into groups, each sharing a common theme:

- intimate relationships
- lack of confidence
- aimless future
- work incompetence
- financial problems.

These themes reflect difficulties in the most important areas of everyday life. Worry is commonly experienced when something is perceived as going wrong in domestic, social or work situations. Research into satisfaction and happiness has shown that a good relationship, a full social life and an enjoyable job are particularly important factors in maintaining happiness. Take a look at Table 2, where various more specific worries relating to these major themes are listed. Then, on a piece of paper, note down any such specific worries that particularly relate to you. See if this exercise helps you identify problem areas of your life. It may be reassuring to understand that these are very common areas of anxiety. It's natural for most people to worry about these major topics at some point in their lives.

In addition to the areas included in the questionnaire, another group of worries often reported is to do with health concerns, often anticipating serious illness or death. In this group we also find worries about accidents. However, these worries are not as common as those mentioned above. In addition, over-concern with one's health is commonly associated with more serious anxiety problems than common or ordinary worry, which this book is about.

Table 2 A worry questionnaire

Relationships

I worry
- that I will lose close friends;
- that I am unattractive to the opposite sex;
- that my family will be angry with me or disapprove of something that I do;
- that I find it difficult to maintain a stable relationship;
- that I am not loved.

Lack of confidence

I worry
- that I cannot be assertive or express my opinions;
- that others will not approve of me;
- that I lack confidence;
- that I might make myself look stupid;
- that I feel insecure.

Aimless future

I worry
- that I'll never achieve my ambitions;
- that I haven't achieved much;
- that my future job prospects are not good;
- that life may have no purpose;
- that I have no concentration.

Work incompetence

I worry
- that I will be late for an appointment;
- that I leave work unfinished;
- that I make mistakes at work;
- that I don't work hard enough;
- that I will not keep my workload up to date.

Financial

I worry
- that my money will run out;
- that I am not able to afford things;
- that financial problems will restrict holidays and travel;
- that my living conditions are inadequate;
- that I can't afford to pay bills.

How do I know if I'm worrying too much?

Earlier, it was suggested that worry is like an alarm system that tells you to deal with a specific problem. Therefore, you should try to see worry as a friend rather than a foe – helpful, not harmful. However, if you find that worry leads to more worry instead of decisions and actions, you might consider what effect this is having on your health. Unnecessary worry is a stress you could probably do without.

Very few studies have looked at the effect of worry on health, though there is some evidence to suggest that too much worry *is* bad for you.

One of the most important findings in recent years has been the role of worry in insomnia. Research shows that one of the main reasons for a sleepless night is worry. Losing sleep is of course in itself unpleasant. However, an irregular pattern of sleep may well disrupt the fragile balance of chemicals that keeps us healthy. Disturbed sleep patterns might lead to hormone-level changes, which in turn make certain types of illness more likely – anything from the common cold to something more serious.

In addition, research into stress has shown that attempting to cope with stressful situations for too long can lead to high blood pressure, which is one of the factors that increase the likelihood of heart attack.

If you are getting more illnesses than usual, then perhaps you are under stress. Are you worrying a lot as a consequence? If so, is it getting you anywhere? Are unwanted thoughts making it difficult for you to get to sleep at night? If so, then you should start to take a closer look at those thoughts. Are they telling you something? Do you need to deal with an outstanding problem?

Now let's consider how we might prepare ourselves for dealing with the problems that cause everyday worry.

2

Preparing to solve your problems

If you are going to be an effective problem-solver, then you need to be working on four areas:

1 Getting some practice. The first section of this chapter explains how important practice is.
2 Learning a 'problem-solving package' – a collection of skills to deal with worry.
3 Developing a positive attitude towards worry – if you see worry as helpful, then you are more likely to use it constructively.
4 Recognizing the early warning signs of worry, so that it will be easier to stop yourself becoming overwhelmed.

Practising skills

As we've said, problems usually underlie worry. To solve problems efficiently, we have to develop problem-solving skills. This takes practice!

This applies to many life skills. For example, many people assume that relaxation is easy, something that happens effortlessly as soon as you sit down. You say to yourself, 'Just relax', but nothing happens. That is because you haven't practised relaxing. Another common example of something that people assume doesn't need practice is dieting. Breaking a diet isn't that serious if you recognize that dieting is a skill. Setbacks can be used to identify areas that need more practice.

It is very common for people to explain their disappointments by blaming themselves. For example, 'I can't relax because I'm a tense person' or 'I'll never lose weight because I haven't got any willpower.' However, unless you've actually practised something again and again, it's impossible to do. You can't attribute your 'failure' to some 'bad' or 'weak' personality trait. You can only really blame yourself for not practising.

So what has all this got to do with worry? Well, the ability to solve everyday problems is one of those things we tend to think of as automatic. In fact, solving everyday problems is a skill that can be easily learnt, and you don't have to be particularly clever.

Skills that are used to solve problems are generally grouped together as **problem-solving packages**. A problem-solving package can be compared to a map or a useful set of instructions. Bear in mind there are usually alternative ways of dealing with a problem. A problem-solving package will help you to work out the various routes.

Changing your attitude towards worry

Although worry can be 'problematic' it isn't really the problem as such. The *real* problem is the situation or person that's bothering us in the first place.

One of the first things you must learn to do is change your attitude to worry, and view it as a helpful mental response that reminds you to deal with a problem. It has to be unpleasant and repetitive, or you wouldn't take any notice of it. Imagine buying an expensive security alarm system that went off very quietly for five seconds!

So, let's start thinking about worry as a useful mental event rather than a burden – something that we can all take advantage of.

Recognizing worry

Worry is an involuntary activity. You don't decide when it begins, and once it has begun it is very difficult to stop. Because worry tends to creep up on you, it's important to recognize it early on. There are two good reasons for this.

First, it's quite easy to get upset by worry, without really being aware of what's happening.

The second reason why it's important to recognize worry early is that it tends to get worse. If you are able to catch it before it really gets going, it might be possible to avoid being overwhelmed, by which time you will probably be too upset to deal with your problems in a constructive way.

Know what your early warning signs are

An important thing to remember is that everybody responds to worry differently. People's responses to worry may include:

- feeling tense;
- feeling more depressed than usual;
- feeling tearful after someone has been rude to you;
- thinking 'I can't cope with this';
- thinking 'I can't face that person any more'.

Keep a diary. Note how you're feeling at different points in the day, and then see if you can find reasons for those feelings. The alarm system is telling you that something is wrong and needs to be dealt with. Don't wait for worry to be intrusive. Try to recognize what your worry is telling you at the earliest convenient moment.

Key points

- First, when you catch yourself worrying, remind yourself that it's letting you know that a problem needs to be dealt with. In this respect, worry can be viewed as a very useful reaction.
- Next, try to sort out what's bothering you early on. It doesn't have to be in detail at this stage – just a rough idea of what you're upset about.
- Lastly, consider whether you're up to sorting things out.

This last point is quite important. If you're coming home from work on a crowded train in the rush hour with a splitting headache, you're probably not going to be able to think straight. Recognize that in stressful situations *you're not at your best*, so put off problem-solving until you're feeling calmer and attempt to distract yourself. Being too wound-up will affect your ability to solve problems. Perhaps after a hot relaxing bath your worries won't seem half as bad.

If you are feeling all right, then you're ready for the first stage of problem-solving – 'problem definition'.

3

How to solve your problems: the problem-solving package

Defining the problem

Defining a problem is surprisingly difficult. Worry will tell you where there is a problem, but it won't necessarily tell you the exact nature of the problem. Everyday problems can be extremely complex. Like an onion, they may have different layers that can be peeled away. Let's take an example.

Laura

Laura was worried about her workload. Although she was working very hard, she kept on making mistakes. But the true source of the problem was her new manager Donald, who was overfamiliar. His tedious amorous advances were beginning to get Laura down. She had stopped going to Donald for advice, and consequently was making some quite serious mistakes.

Always think carefully about what is bothering you. A good way to find out is to talk things over with a friend. There's good evidence to suggest that the more you do this the better you feel. Perhaps discussing things helps people get to the bottom of what's troubling them. In other words, they are able to define their problem more accurately, which in turn helps them to deal with it more effectively when the time comes.

You may well be worried about more than one thing. In this case you will have to define several problems. Try to see where one problem ends and another begins. You can do this by making a list.

Don't attempt to solve all your problems at once. The best thing to do is take them one at a time. This means that you will have to put some worries on hold. This is going to be difficult, as the whole purpose of worry seems to be to capture your attention. However, by postponing addressing some problems, you will be able to deal with others more efficiently. You will really be able to concentrate on the problem in hand. By the time you get around to dealing with postponed problems, you should be less stressed, having disposed of others already.

Make use of distraction. If you're likely to spend a whole evening worrying about problems that you intend to deal with but can't at present, then arrange to go out. An exciting film, or dinner with friends, might take your mind off things. Provided you are doing something about at least one of your problems, then you can afford to leave the others alone for a short while. However, don't forget that worry cannot really be ignored; distracting yourself can only ever be a stopgap measure. Eventually, each problem will have to be dealt with, or worry will continue.

Solve your easiest problems first. Choose one that you can actually do something about. There are some things in life that you simply can't change.

Thinking up solutions (brainstorming)

After defining the source of your worry, the next thing to do is to ask yourself, 'What can I do about it?' Usually, if you are presented with a problem, it is possible to think of more than one solution – a process sometimes called brainstorming. The more choice you have, then the more chance you have of selecting a way of coping that is just right for you.

Before you start brainstorming there are a couple of things you should try to remember. The first is to suspend judgement. What this means is: don't be too self-critical. If you think up a way of dealing with a problem, then make a note of it, whatever it is. We can sort out the good ideas from the bad ones later. At this stage, the important thing is to stop yourself from dismissing ideas before you've given them a fair chance. Many people lack confidence in their own ability to cope with problems. Writing down as many ideas as you can will help you to get over a self-confidence barrier.

Many people have a tendency to say 'Yes, but . . .' when presented with a possible solution. One of the good things about brainstorming is that it will help you to overcome this tendency. If you say 'Yes, but . . .' too soon, you will never get the chance to evaluate your ideas fully. An incidental point to remember is that we are all sometimes reluctant to deal with our problems. After all, dealing with a problem often involves effort and, under some circumstances, confrontation. It might seem easier in the short term to avoid a particular problem than to deal with it. However, most problems don't solve themselves, and as long as we are aware of them they are likely to be a source of nagging worry.

Brainstorming will help you to get out of the habit of saying 'Yes, but . . .' Remember: there is plenty of time available in which to evaluate your ideas. So suspend your judgement and let the ideas come thick and fast!

Making decisions: weighing up the pros and cons

The next stage of problem-solving is deciding what to do. A good way to start doing this is to list the pros and cons associated with each solution to your problem, as shown in Table 3.

Sue

Sue had been a laboratory technician in a hospital for the past five years, but felt bored and trapped, and had begun worrying about her future. 'What am I doing with my life?'

Sue had once been a voluntary counsellor at an advice centre and had enjoyed it very much. So one possible solution to her frustrations at work was to become a professional counsellor, an idea she found very appealing. Her second solution was to try to make her job as a laboratory technician more active and interesting.

We can see from Table 3 that there are more pros than cons associated with becoming a counsellor, whereas there are more cons than pros associated with taking a more active role at work. It would seem, then, that Sue would be better off changing her job.

However, just counting up pros and cons can be misleading. All pros are not equally advantageous, and not all cons are equally problematic. For example, let us imagine an individual who is evaluating the merits

Table 3 Sue's solutions

Solution one: Career change?

Pros	Cons
I'll really enjoy being a counsellor.	I'll have to get a new qualification.
I might be able to work from home: no long journeys on the train!	If I become self-employed, this will be risky. What if nobody comes to see me?
I wouldn't have to use the computer anymore. I always find that difficult.	If I have to study again, I'll have to do a part-time course. This will damage my social life.
When I'm qualified, I might have more free time.	

Solution two: Taking a more active role?

Pros	Cons
I might get a pay rise.	I'll have to be more forceful. This is quite difficult in my department.
My life won't be disrupted.	I'll have to work a lot harder.
	I may be asked to give talks on special topics. I hate talking in public.
	I'll have to see a lot more of the head of the department. We never get on very well.

of two jobs. In the pros column of the first job the following is written: 'I will double my income.' However, in the pros column of the second job we find: 'I will be able to have an extra five-minute tea break.' Clearly, the pro relating to the first job (doubled income) is considerably more important than the pro relating to the second job (additional tea break).

A way of getting around this problem is by placing a number, called a weighting, next to each pro and each con. The weighting represents how important each statement is. It's usually a good idea to do this by picking a number between 1 and 10. There is a slight limitation here, in that your most important item cannot be rated as more than ten times as important as your least important item. Because of this, some people find it easier to rate items using a wider range, say between 1 and 50. However, there are no hard and fast rules: choose a scale that you feel comfortable with. Table 4 shows what Sue's lists will look like with weightings included.

Bear in mind that Table 4 is a very crude example of a list of pros and cons. When making a serious career decision, it is not always possible to reduce the advantages and disadvantages in this way. A pros and cons list is a way of helping you to decide which potential solution to choose. A number of books give the impression that this technique is a powerful method of assisting decision-making, but perhaps this is over-optimistic. A more sensible view is that making a list of good and bad consequences helps you to clarify issues associated with a particular decision.

Some people find that after adding up the pros and cons the numbers tell them that a first solution is better than a second solution. However, they still feel reluctant to go ahead with their first solution. There are a number of ways of looking at such an outcome. Sometimes we just don't feel right about a particular decision, even when the evidence is in favour of it. Under these circumstances it's a good idea to talk things over with someone in order to get to the

Table 4 Sue's scores

Solution one: Career change?

Pros		Cons	
I'll really enjoy being a counsellor.	8	I'll have to get a new qualification.	3
I might be able to work from home: no long journeys on the train!	5	If I become self-employed, this will be risky. What if nobody comes to see me?	7
I wouldn't have to use the computer anymore. I always find that difficult.	3	If I have to study again, I'll have to do a part-time course. This will damage my social life.	5
When I'm qualified I might have more free time.	7		
TOTAL	**23**		**15**

If we add up the weightings, we find that the total for pros is 23, whereas the total for cons is 15. The difference between 23 and 15 is 8, in favour of pros. In other words, there are more good things associated with becoming a counsellor than bad things.

Solution two: Taking a more active role?

Pros		Cons	
I might get a pay rise.	4	I'll to have be more forceful. This is quite difficult in my department.	7
My life won't be disrupted.	7	I'll have to work a lot harder.	6
		I may be asked to give talks on special topics. I hate talking in public.	5
		I'll have to see a lot more of the head of the department. We never get on very well.	7
TOTAL	**11**		**25**

The difference between 11 and 25 is 14, in favour of cons. This means that there are more drawbacks associated with trying to take a more active role in the department than there are good things. Clearly, the best decision for Sue is to change career. This appears to be the best plan.

bottom of those reservations. Perhaps your lists are incomplete, in that there are some things that need to be written down that you've missed out. On the other hand, perhaps the problem is so complex that it just cannot be reduced to a list of 'for' and 'against' items. Remember: listing pros and cons is simply a helpful way of clarifying issues. Feeling uncomfortable about the outcome of a particular set of pros and cons might be a necessary step towards uncovering a deeper problem. Let's take another example.

Alice

Alice was offered two jobs. The first was a well-paid management position in a large department store fairly close to her home. The second wasn't so well paid, and involved working as a secretary in the office of an interior design company. After doing a pros and cons analysis she wasn't surprised to find that there were many more advantages associated with taking up the management job. However, she just didn't feel right. Although there would be more money, more responsibility and good promotion prospects if she took the management job, she just didn't want to do it. Money wasn't really her priority. She had always been interested in design, and would have perhaps gone to a design college had her parents not bullied her into taking business studies. Her pros and cons analysis reflected more of what her husband and family wanted her to do than what she wanted to do herself. Her real inclination was to take the secretarial post, so that she could see how a design company worked.

When choosing between options, you have to ask yourself not only 'What do I want?' but also 'What do I *really* want?' This is because our *real* needs aren't always easy to recognize. Some psychologists and counsellors ask their clients to make a distinction between **self** and

self-concept. The self is 'you', who you really are. The self-concept is the 'you' that owes much to the expectations and values of others. As we develop as people, we often accept ideas and values that have very little to do with us. When we make decisions, we may feel uncomfortable because the decision has been influenced by our self-concept, more than our true self.

When you make a decision, ask: 'Why do I want to do this?' Is it because you want to do it? Or is it because you think it is the correct and proper thing to do? If so, correct and proper by whose standards? Yours? Or your parents'? If you have a voice in your head saying that you 'should' solve your problem this way, or that you 'ought to' solve your problem that way, then question it!

There is in fact very little in this life that you 'should' or 'ought to' do. Statements worded in this way are probably closer to your parents' or somebody else's wishes than to yours. If you use a pros and cons analysis and are still feeling unsure, then reconsider how you weighted the pros and cons. Do the values reflect your feelings, or someone else's?

If we become sensitive to our true feelings, then this might have a dramatic effect on how we view decisions. We might choose to give up striving to achieve something, because when we look at the achievement we see it has more to do with other people's wishes than our own. Giving up, under these circumstances, is a successful decision.

This is not only true of 'giving up' decisions, it is also true of 'go-for-it' decisions. Recognizing what you want for yourself might have the effect of inspiring you to consider choices that you previously failed to acknowledge. Perhaps your parents and other significant people in your life have always discouraged you from taking certain types of decision.

Earlier, we said that a pros and cons analysis might not work because the lists were incomplete. However, it might be the case that there is sufficient evidence available for you to make a decision but you still can't choose. This is a major problem for worriers!

4

Learning to make
quicker decisions

Swifter decision-making is likely to reduce the amount of time you spend worrying. Now, if you are an inveterate worrier, you are likely to have some fairly strong beliefs about quick decisions. You will probably be naturally cautious, and feel that a quick decision means taking unnecessary risks. 'More haste, less speed.' But this proverb, like all proverbs, tells the truth, but not the whole truth! Of course making hasty decisions and rushing into things is a bad idea. However, this doesn't mean that making a quick decision is always wrong. Further, if you have defined your problem carefully and considered the pros and cons associated with several ways of coping, you can hardly be accused of rushing into something.

We have seen that worriers often demand more evidence than is readily available, in an attempt to be absolutely sure that they are doing the right thing. If you do not accept such evidence as is available, you will be paralysed by indecision. You will find yourself going over the same things again and again, in an effort to be absolutely sure that what you are about to do is correct.

Life would be considerably easier if we could predict the future. The popularity of astrology columns in magazines and newspapers gives us some idea of how powerful this 'need to know' actually is. Even the most rational people will sometimes have a quick look at their 'stars'. Astrology has remained popular because, for many people, living with uncertainty is quite difficult. Astrology can be comforting, in that it appears to take away some of that uncertainty.

Unfortunately, it really is impossible to know the future, whatever we might want to believe. When we select a coping strategy, we are simply choosing to do something that, to the best of our knowledge, has a good chance of achieving a desired goal. All decisions are risky decisions in that sense. There is no such thing as a decision that has no risk attached to it. Going down the road to buy a loaf of bread could be seen as a highly risky business: you might get run over! The baker might decide to shoot you! An aeroplane might crash on your head! It is always possible to think of things that can go wrong. These examples are admittedly bizarre; however, worriers can delay decision-making because of this kind of thinking. A worrier who has defined a problem might know exactly which options are available, but feel that there isn't enough evidence favouring one in particular.

So how do we go about making quicker decisions?

First, become accustomed to taking *sensible risks*. Although we cannot know with absolute certainty what is going to happen, we all have enough life experience to have a pretty good guess. For our purposes, exact knowledge is unnecessary.

Start by making quicker decisions about things where the consequences are not too serious either way. You needn't wait for a problem to do this. You can make quicker decisions about choosing between pleasant options, such as which of two books to buy.

Do a quick pros and cons analysis of each in your head, then just go ahead and buy one. Remember: even if the book you buy turns out to be less enjoyable than you thought, does it really matter? Worriers have a habit of turning minor problems into major catastrophes. You can always buy the other book some other time!

The above example is interesting in that it shows how worriers can find something to worry about in the least threatening situations. The worrier will be able to make the situation unpleasant by thinking about failing to make the best possible choice, instead of thinking: 'I'll enjoy both of them to some extent, whichever one I buy, so I may as well buy this one.'

After you have practised making simple decisions more swiftly, have a go at harder ones. You might give yourself a deadline, and stick to it, even if you're still unsure or a little uncomfortable.

Key points

- Worry will fill up the time between recognizing a threat or problem, and dealing with it.
- The quicker you deal with your problem, the less time you will spend worrying.
- There is never enough evidence available to ensure that your decision is absolutely right; there are always risks.
- If you have defined your problem carefully and evaluated ways of coping with that problem, you are not being rash or hasty.
- Finally, if you have begun to act on the basis of one of your decisions, see it through. All decisions have pros and cons. Don't focus on the cons! It is easy to regret making a decision if you only think about

associated drawbacks. Always remind yourself of the advantages!

Being realistic

Once you have generated a number of coping strategies, it is important to be realistic. Don't attempt to solve a problem in a way that might be beyond your capabilities. Although it isn't a good idea to limit yourself, neither is it a good idea to attempt to solve a problem in a way to which you are not suited. We all have limitations.

For some people, failure becomes habitual. Indeed, setting unrealistic goals and constantly failing can be reassuring. If you know that you are going to fail, the world is less unpredictable. Perhaps more importantly, if you know that you are going to fail, you can avoid all the effort involved in dealing with a troublesome situation.

Some people use their own 'incompetence' and 'helplessness' as a manipulative tool. The underlying assumption is: 'If I can't do it, then somebody else will have to do it for me.' Sadly, not all of our problems can be shifted on to the shoulders of others. So do be careful. If you find that you are attracted to ways of solving problems that have never proved effective for you in the past, then think again. Try to select a coping strategy that you might have used successfully before. If you can't think of one, then make a list of things that you're good at. Would any of these skills be useful when attempting to solve your problem? Do they correspond with the demands of the coping strategy you have selected?

If you don't have much self-confidence, then you probably don't think you have many skills to fall back on. You might, for example, think that you're not very clever. However, being clever isn't all that important. You might be a very warm person. As it happens, being warm is a skill that a lot of so-called clever people haven't acquired! Being warm might be a really important characteristic for the success of a particular coping strategy. So don't adopt a narrow view of what constitutes a skill. You probably have a wealth of skills, but as yet don't regard them as such.

Key points

So when attempting to select a solution to your problem, you could do the following:

- First, use a pros and cons analysis to clarify issues and sort out which strategy will give you the best possible outcome.
- Second, consider how well equipped you are. By all means take up a difficult challenge, but by the same token, don't attempt to solve a problem that demands skills you do not have, or are unlikely to acquire.
- Third, act on your decision. Remind yourself that unless you solve your problem, you will keep on experiencing worry. Turn your worry into actions as soon as possible.

Problem-solving stages

You might find thinking about your problems easier when prompted with questions. So you might choose to make a list of questions like that shown in Table 5 (overleaf), which reflect the stages of problem-solving.

Table 5 Problem-solving stages

- What am I worried about?
- What do I want to happen?
- What can I do to make it happen?
- What is actually likely to happen?
- What is my decision?

And after you have implemented your coping strategy:

- Did it work?

The great advantage of problem-solving approaches is that they allow you to break problems down in a systematic way. It is much easier to deal with a problem in small steps that follow on logically from each other than to deal with a problem in one go. Everyday problems can often feel as though they are about to get 'out of control'. Problem-solving is a way you can regain control over your life and re-establish some sort of order.

Evaluation

The final stage in problem-solving is evaluating your progress. Did the coping strategy you selected deal with the problem? If the answer is yes, then well done. Give yourself a pat on the back, or an immediate treat. If you are not used to treating yourself, then make a reward menu, such as going to the cinema or buying some new clothes. When you have successfully resolved a problem, indulge yourself! Rewards don't have to be big. A book or magazine might be sufficient. The main thing is to acknowledge your own success.

If your coping strategy has failed, so what? It really isn't the end of the world. You can always have another go. Go back to your list of alternative ways of dealing with the problem – that is, the list compiled after brain-storming – and select another strategy. If this doesn't seem right, then you can always go right back to the beginning, the problem-definition stage, and redefine your problem. As we said earlier, it is easy to confuse problems.

Also, remember that some things look easier to do on paper than they are in real life.

As we said earlier, problem-solving is a skill. You may find that before you can deal with worrying problems, you need a great deal of practice. Don't be discouraged by setbacks. Don't fall into the trap of thinking that one setback means that you will always fail. Although setbacks are upsetting, don't allow them to put you off having another go. We have already stressed that it is impossible to know the future. Treat each new attempt to solve your problem as if it is the first.

5

Coping with setbacks

Thoughts and feelings: a close relationship

The distinction between people who think and people who feel is very misleading. Everybody has thoughts, and everybody has feelings. In fact, the two are very closely related. It is even possible to suggest that thinking happy or sad thoughts can change our mood for better or for worse.

Negative thinking

We have already said that worriers tend to take a negative view of things. This is especially true when worriers view their own personalities. If you look at the worry items shown in Table 2, you will see that many of them reflect low levels of self-confidence.

It would appear that negative thinking has a powerful effect on mood. When people have difficulty coping, thoughts like 'I'm worthless' or 'I'm useless' pop into their minds automatically. If you do anything for long enough it will become automatic. For example, most people don't have to think about changing gear when they are driving. They simply do it automatically. When people get into the habit of thinking negatively about themselves, they do so with the same degree of automation. Derogatory remarks come to mind so easily that half the time they don't even realize what they're thinking. They feel sad, but don't see the connection between their thoughts and the way they feel.

However, psychologists and psychiatrists have found that these thoughts can be changed. Once an individual becomes aware of how thoughts can influence feelings, then he or she can learn to identify negative thoughts. Once negative thoughts have been identified, it is then possible to practise replacing them with more appropriate thoughts. This kind of treatment has become known as **cognitive therapy** or **cognitive behavioural therapy (CBT)**, and is extremely helpful to those suffering from depression. Results show that cognitive therapy makes people less inclined to take a negative view of things, and therefore more able to deal with their problems.

At this point you might want to ask the question: 'Why should you replace negative thoughts if they are accurate?' The answer is, you shouldn't. A realistic evaluation of a problem may well be negative. However, psychologists have shown that people who think negatively are generally anything but realistic. The thoughts that they have are biased in favour of a negative view. In addition, negative thoughts are often treated mistakenly as facts. Negative thinkers rarely consider how accurate their automatic thoughts are. Most negative thoughts should be treated not as facts, but as possible facts that have to be tested. When we get a negative thought we should ask ourselves, 'Is this really true?'

The process of self-questioning is very important. Usually, we don't believe everything we're told. If we did, then we could all be easily misled by the tabloids into believing, for example, that Elvis Presley is currently alive and well in Grimsby, and Second World War bombers can be found on the moon! Unfortunately, most people look at their own thoughts less critically than they do the Sunday papers. Sometimes our own thoughts are equally absurd! During cognitive therapy, most people are surprised to find that a little time spent challenging negative thoughts will reveal dramatic inaccuracies.

Earlier it was said that negative thoughts can be replaced with more appropriate thoughts – that is, more *realistic*, not necessarily more positive, thoughts. So-called 'positive thinking' can be as unhelpful as negative thinking. It often involves replacing one unrealistic thought with a different kind of unrealistic thought. If you keep saying to yourself, 'Everything will be all right', when there is no good reason to think that things *will* be all right, then such a thought will be entirely inappropriate. Attempting to look on the bright side when things are going wrong all around you will do you no good at all. Negative thoughts must always be replaced with realistic thoughts. The good news is that most realistic thoughts are more optimistic than negative thoughts, and considerably less rigid.

Key points

- Negative thoughts have to be carefully evaluated.
- They are often automatic and, because of this, wrong.
- However, because we treat them as facts, they can make us feel bad about ourselves and the world we live in.
- Negative thoughts can be changed to realistic thoughts. These are often more optimistic!

Negative thinking and problem-solving

Make a clear distinction in your mind between setbacks and failures. If you cannot solve a particular problem, then must you call your attempt a failure? It would be more useful to see early difficulties as a temporary setback – then you are more likely to renew your efforts. For example, if you break a diet it doesn't mean that the diet has failed at all. You can always have another go.

The word 'setback' is less final than 'failure'. Try to use it more often. After a setback, you may find that the next coping strategy you choose will work really well.

Every time you get a negative thought, you must try to challenge it rationally, if you can. Fortunately, negative thoughts are not that difficult to detect. In addition, they can conveniently be grouped under headings.

Below we list five types of negative thought.

Black-and-white thinking

Example: If I can't do problem-solving perfectly, then I may as well give up!

A black-and-white thinker sees things in terms of all or nothing. Something must be either all good or totally bad. Problem-solving has to be accomplished to a high standard, or it's not worth bothering with. You are either on a diet or off a diet. Eating a chocolate biscuit means that you are 'off' and have therefore failed.

This type of thinking is highly unproductive. If you have unrealistic expectations then you are going to set yourself up for failure. It is impossible to solve problems perfectly after one or two attempts. There will always be something that could have been done better. Remember: progress depends on practice.

Improvements may be very gradual, but these small improvements will add up over time, perhaps even over several weeks or months. So don't expect too much, too soon.

Making a little progress really is better than none at all. If you reject problem-solving because it doesn't deliver the goods immediately, then you might fail to see how tackling your problem has in fact got you one step closer to a less worry-filled life.

If you tend to think in black-and-white terms, remember to challenge yourself. Is this type of negative thought true? If you can't do problem-solving perfectly, does it really mean there are no advantages? Why can't you get better at problem-solving gradually?

Perhaps you could prepare some statements that you can read whenever you find yourself indulging in black-and-white thinking. For example:

> Although I didn't solve my problem very effectively, I did feel more in control of my worry.

or

> Maybe I could have defined my problem more accurately. The fact is, I know where I'm going wrong now, and next time I'll be able to do it better.

Overgeneralization

Example: Problem-solving didn't work now, so why should it ever work?

Overgeneralization is drawing sweeping conclusions on the basis of a single event. We often do this by making false connections. For example, you might think that because you can't play tennis very well, you probably can't play squash very well either. In fact the two games are very different, and it's quite easy to be a good squash player without being good at tennis!

Another way we can overgeneralize is by thinking that one poor performance predicts another. Everybody has off days. All sorts of things might reduce our efficiency. Perhaps you are feeling too tense. Perhaps you are too tired. Perhaps there's too much noise outside. The important thing to remember is that if something goes wrong once, it doesn't mean that it will *always* go wrong.

The world is full of examples of failures preceding successes. Have you ever listened to cars starting on a cold morning? The first turn of the ignition key will usually fail to start the car. Does that mean the car will never start? Of course not. After anything between two and twenty turns you will hear the engine ticking over. For the driver, persistent effort has paid off. He or she will be able to get to work on time. In other words, the first attempts at starting the car were setbacks, not failures.

If you think that you overgeneralize, then be prepared to challenge your thoughts. Is it really true that because you never did well at school, you will never be clever enough to deal with your problems? Why should today's disappointments stop you from succeeding tomorrow? Are there any good reasons why you should think in this way?

You might find preparing replacement thoughts like the following helpful, if you overgeneralize:

Problem-solving didn't work as well as I thought. Maybe I should relax and try again later.

or

Just because things went wrong today doesn't mean they won't work out tomorrow.

Blaming yourself

Example: It all went wrong because of me!

When things go wrong we often blame ourselves. This is because sometimes it's the easiest thing to do. Human beings are always trying to work out why things happen. If something goes wrong and there isn't an obvious reason why, then we will look for someone to blame. If there isn't anybody around to blame, we are likely to blame ourselves.

This need to accuse is particularly evident in the newspapers, especially after a disaster. In most cases it is extremely difficult to prove that someone is blameworthy. When something like a disaster occurs, this is usually because a number of small things have been adding up. The same applies to our personal lives. If something goes wrong, it might be because a whole series of events has been leading up to it. Most of these events will probably be out of our control. Therefore it is senseless to indulge in self-blame.

If you cannot solve problems efficiently, don't leap to the conclusion that you are lazy or negligent. Of course, it is possible that you are being lazy and negligent! However, such an evaluation is likely to be incorrect if you are a negative thinker. It is more likely that you are blaming yourself for a setback because that is what you usually do. A closer examination of the circumstances that led up to your setback might reveal the effects of factors out of your control.

If you feel that you haven't been very good at problem-solving, then try to establish why. Maybe you haven't put much effort into it, but this lack of commitment might be because of some other problem. Maybe you've only just got over the flu or are feeling tired or premenstrual, in which case is it really your fault? If you make mistakes because you are upset, then ask yourself why you are upset. Perhaps somebody was rude to you this morning. Was that your fault? If you habitually blame yourself, then it is time to break the habit. A close look at your mistakes will most probably reveal that some causes have little, if anything, to do with you. You cannot accept the blame for things that you cannot do anything about.

We have said before that problem-solving involves using a collection of skills. If you get these skills wrong occasionally, you may need more practice. Getting the skills wrong is not the same as *being* wrong. When things go wrong, get out of the habit of calling yourself names like 'stupid' or 'useless'. It is important to pre-serve a sense of self-worth and self-respect. Even if you do make mistakes sometimes, that does not mean that you are a worthless person!

Try to replace your blaming thoughts with more constructive statements. For example:

> It was impossible for me to have known that that would happen – I did my best.

or

> Just because things went wrong this time doesn't mean that I'm stupid.

Predicting the future

Example: It's sure to go wrong!
We all make predictions all the time. Although you probably don't think of it as predicting, every time you leave your house or flat to go shopping you are in fact making several predictions. The most important one is that the shops will be open. A second important prediction might be that the shops will have what

you want to buy. However, even simple predictions like this are sometimes incorrect. We often find shops unexpectedly closed. Or perhaps they have sold out of the commodities we require.

At best, we only ever have a rough idea of what is going to happen in the future.

If you are a negative thinker, then most of your predictions will favour negative outcomes. In addition, you will have a tendency to treat these negative predictions as facts. Such predictions are clearly biased.

If you have already predicted that 'problem-solving won't stop me worrying', then challenge that prediction. How can you be so sure? A more realistic prediction would be that 'problem-solving may or may not stop me worrying'. This latter prediction is far more realistic. It acknowledges the fact that you are not psychic and cannot look into the future! Also, unlike the former prediction, it recognizes the possibility of things turning out all right, as well as going wrong.

Finally, a word should be said about 'mind-reading'. This is when we predict what other people are thinking, and how they will react. As with predicting the future, we know that some things are more likely than others. Our best friend is less likely to hit us than our worst enemy. However, we should never assume that we know what's going on in somebody else's head. If you have a tendency to think the worst, then always try to examine the evidence for and against your predictions. Some alternative thoughts that might replace your negative predictions are:

> I keep thinking things won't work out – but in fact it's impossible to predict the future.

or

> I keep on predicting how other people will react –
> but it's impossible to say: I'm not a mind-reader.

Dismissing successes

Example: I solved this problem, but so what!

Last of all, don't dismiss your successes. If you solve one problem, then good for you. That means you can solve another, and another after that. The more problems you solve, the less you will have to worry about. You can get out of the habit of dismissing your successes by rewarding yourself. Needless to say, if you succeed, reward yourself.

Remember: when you do solve a problem, it really does mean something.

- It means that you have taken control of your life.
- It means that you are less vulnerable to worry, and therefore less likely to suffer the consequences, like sleepless nights.
- In the long term, this means you will be a healthier, fitter person.
- When you manage to solve a problem, you will be able to concentrate more on the things you enjoy.
- Finally, it means that you will be better equipped the next time a problem develops in your life.

Remind yourself that problem-solving is an achievement that deserves rewarding. Perhaps you could prepare statements like the following:

> Because I solved my problem, I haven't worried for a week. That's quite an achievement.

or

> Well done! I solved the problem: I'll go to the cinema tonight as a reward.

If you constantly challenge negative thoughts and look for facts that disprove them, you will soon learn that negative thinking is not only unhelpful, but largely misleading. The future is not always as bleak as you might think.

6

When the worry won't stop

This is not pessimistic! Although it happens quite rarely, most people will at one time or another be forced to admit that a situation or circumstance is simply uncontrollable. However, there are ways of dealing with problems that seem insoluble.

What to do if you still need more practice!

Let's assume that although you have been trying to solve problems regularly, your efforts have been unsuccessful. For the sake of making the difficulty explicit, let's say that when trying to define a problem, you are always unable to trace the worry back to a single cause. This results in the selection of inappropriate coping strategies and continued worry. What can be done under these circumstances?

- Remind yourself that practice will eventually improve your problem-solving skills. Although you find problem definition hard today, this might not be the case tomorrow.
- Remind yourself of the distinction between setbacks and failure, and then identify any negative thoughts you might have experienced.
- If you notice that you have been overgeneralizing or perhaps trying to predict the future (see Chapter 5), then challenge these thoughts and replace them with more realistic thoughts.

- Finally, when you are in a relaxed frame of mind, have another go at defining the problem.

Although the above suggestions might help you to cope with a temporary setback, they do not reduce the impact of your existing problem or problems. You are still worrying, and as yet are unsure if your next attempt at problem-solving will have the desired effect. Under these circumstances, what can you do?

First, recognize that worry catastrophizes (see p. 1). If you have been worrying a great deal, then it is quite possible that the disasters you anticipate will never actually happen. Ask yourself the following questions:

- How many people do I know who have been unable to survive a relationship problem?
- How many people do I know who simply couldn't cope with life because they lacked confidence?
- How many people do I know who have never achieved a single ambition?
- How many people do I know who have lost their jobs because they made too many mistakes?
- Finally, how many people do I know who have found themselves in serious trouble – for example, prison – because of financial problems?

Unless you have an extremely unlucky group of friends, the answer to most if not all of the above questions will be few or none! The worst very rarely happens. Even if we can't solve our problems, unpleasant consequences are rarely as catastrophic as we imagine. Coping with a real bad outcome is sometimes easier than coping with an imagined one. If you can't solve your problems yet, then remind yourself that worry can turn molehills into mountains.

Key points

- If you're finding it difficult to solve problems, then remind yourself that more effort will probably be a worthwhile investment.
- Second, remind yourself that worry catastrophizes. Most of the disasters that you imagine simply won't happen.
- Finally, remember that even if the worst does happen, the consequences might not be as terrible as you anticipate.

Problems that can't be solved

Some things that make us worry we can do nothing about. Even if we are efficient problem-solvers, situations occur that we cannot change. This kind of insoluble problem is quite different from those discussed in the last section. A problem that can be solved by perseverance is somehow less daunting than a problem that appears totally resistant to resolution. When we know that we can't solve a problem whatever we do, this can be quite depressing. We feel that we cannot exercise any control over our lives.

Ageing and dying are two obvious examples of insoluble problems, though not all insoluble problems are as dramatic. For example, psychologists and psychiatrists have found that it is very difficult to stop people being jealous. Another common example of an insoluble problem can be physical illness.

People often report worrying quite a lot about social and political problems. Although these can be solved by the slow process of political change, desired changes will not happen overnight. Further, the threat of terrorism, starvation in the Global South and climate change will be with us for some time to come. But we can stop treating the world as a problem, and treat our emotions as a problem instead. Even when we face inevitabilities, we are not totally powerless. We can still try to change ourselves.

This distinction between changing the world and changing our *response* to the world is an important one. Psychologists have called these two ways of coping **problem-focused coping** and **emotion-focused coping**.

Problem-focused coping is what happens when you tackle the problem at source. That is, you change your circumstances by doing something different.

When doing something different will have no effect on the problem, then it is best to endorse an emotion-focused coping strategy. Instead of attempting to change the world, you must attempt to change the way you are reacting to the world. So, although you may not be able to do anything about an illness, you can still try to alter the way you feel about it. If you are frightened, you might try to turn that fear into peaceful resignation.

When you find that problem-solving isn't working, then reconsider the nature of your problem. Can you really do anything about it? The answer to this question is extremely important. If you decide you can do something about it when in fact you can't, then you may find yourself banging your head against a brick wall. Attempting to solve an insoluble problem can be upsetting and frustrating. If you are worrying over a problem that you cannot seem to solve, then re-evaluate your approach. Perhaps problem-focused coping should be abandoned in favour of emotion-focused coping. Remember: we are not abandoning problem-solving.

Emotion-focused coping is simply a different sort of problem-solving, in which the problem is defined in terms of an emotional reaction. How then might we change our emotional responses?

The relationship between the individual and his or her emotions is a complicated one. Therefore it would be misleading to suggest that changing our emotional response is easy. We must consider not only the intensity of an emotional reaction, but also the strengths and weaknesses of the person dealing with that reaction.

Denial Sometimes the best thing to do is to avoid thinking about very upsetting problems. Psychologists call this reaction 'denial'. It can be very effective. Indeed, there is evidence to suggest that some people suffering from very serious illnesses fare better when they are able to deny their problem. In addition, recent research has shown that people who have experienced really terrible things in the past – such as concentration camps – are able to lead happier lives if they ignore their bad thoughts.

Of course, learning to ignore bad thoughts isn't easy. Not everybody can develop this skill. Try denial and see if it works for you. If ignoring your bad thoughts makes life easier, then try to improve this skill. If you find that it makes matters worse, then obviously it would be foolish to continue using this strategy.

Distraction As suggested earlier, watch a film; or see friends or relatives.

You can face an unavoidable problem by thinking about it yourself, or perhaps talking over the implications with other people. A friend's voice, the touch of another's hand or an expression of affection can provide much-needed support in these circumstances. It's always easier to face a problem if you can share your feelings about it with someone else. Try to be honest. Don't keep your feelings bottled up or try to put on a brave face. If you want to cry, then go ahead and cry. If you're frightened, then say so. In this way, you will be able to get a clear view of how you are feeling. Sometimes it is necessary to let things out, if change is to take place.

Worry and anxiety

Sometimes worry can be part of a more serious problem, such as anxiety. In fact, there are a whole group of problems that are related in some way to the experience of anxiety. For example, phobias, sudden panics and obsessions are all described as anxiety problems.

Briefly, one example of an anxiety problem is **generalized anxiety disorder (GAD)**. Sometimes also described as 'free-floating anxiety', this is a problem strongly associated with worry.

People who suffer from generalized anxiety are usually very tense, and worry excessively. Sweating, flushing, a pounding heart and upset stomach are frequently experienced, often accompanied by worries about losing control in a public place, having a heart attack or becoming fatally ill.

These symptoms – upsetting thoughts and unpleasant bodily sensations – can appear without any apparent cause. Because the symptoms are sometimes difficult to account for, the anxious person is often treated unsympathetically at home. Many people suffering from generalized anxiety are perfectly aware that many of their worries appear strange to other people.

However, this recognition has no effect on the amount of worry experienced. Misfortunes continue to be anticipated even if they never actually happen.

If generalized anxiety becomes too difficult to live with, then it is advisable to seek help. This usually means a visit to the family doctor, who may recommend talking therapies such as counselling or cognitive behavioural therapy. CBT helps you identify unhelpful and unrealistic beliefs and behaviour, and replace them with more helpful and realistic ones. Effective relaxation techniques may also be suggested. Your GP can also offer medication. The options should be discussed in detail and, depending on your symptoms, include selective serotonin reuptake inhibitors (SSRIs), antidepressants that increase the level of the chemical serotonin in your brain, and sometimes, as a short-term measure, tranquillizers, usually one of a group of drugs called the benzodiazepines. Although tranquillizers can be helpful in the short term, they are usually unhelpful and definitely addictive if taken for an extended period of time. A number of side effects are associated with tranquillizers, including severe headaches and nausea. However, the most serious problem by far with benzodiazepines is that they are addictive, and this can be both distressing in itself and difficult to overcome. For this reason, the National Institute for Health and Care Excellence (NICE) strongly advises against their use except in crisis, while the Royal College of GPs also advises great care in prescribing such drugs. An estimated 1.5 million people in the UK are addicted to benzodiazepines, often older people as a result of over-prescribing decades ago.

Ideally, a general practitioner will refer anxiety patients through the NHS for treatment with a clinical psychologist. Most clinical psychologists help people to manage their worries and anxiety by using something called **anxiety management training**, which usually involves learning about relaxation, discussing worries in some detail, and also learning to face particular situations if you find that they are associated with increased levels of anxiety. Anxiety management training can be given to individual patients, or to patients attending a clinic in small groups. If you think that you are suffering from generalized anxiety and think you might have to see a clinical psychologist, remember: this does not mean that you are mad, mentally ill or sick. Because you are not suffering from a disease or illness you will not receive drugs or medication.

Clinical psychologists tend to treat anxiety as a normal emotional response. After all, it can be very useful. If you climb to the top of a ladder, you will probably experience some mild anxiety. This alerts you to the potential danger of falling off and you exercise appropriate caution; if you were totally relaxed in this situation, then you might stop taking care. Clearly, this would increase your chances of having a serious accident. Psychologists don't try to get rid of anxiety, because anxiety is a normal emotional response, but only attempt to reduce levels of anxiety so that life can go on without unnecessary disruptions.

Conclusions

In this chapter we have considered worries that cannot be dealt with by problem-solving. However, let us end on an optimistic note. There are few problems that you will be able to do nothing about. If you are having trouble dealing with problems because you need more practice at problem-solving, then it will only be a matter of time before your skills improve to the extent that worry is reduced. If your problem is genuinely insoluble, then we have mentioned the idea of emotion-focused coping. Although you might not be able to solve the problem that's making you worry, you might be able to change the way you feel about it. If this change is successful, you will probably worry less. Finally, although you may find worry difficult to deal with if it is part of an anxiety problem, that does not mean that you will never be able to deal with it. If you see a clinical psychologist, then you will be taught a number of skills that will help you to reduce levels of anxiety and the amount you worry.

The circumstances outlined above are exceptional. Virtually all the worries you are likely to have will be related to everyday life problems, which can be solved using problem-solving techniques. By systematically analysing your problems, you will be able to generate solutions capable of resolving them. Armed with a systematic approach, you will be able to use worry constructively. Hopefully, after reading this book, you will see worry as helpful rather than harmful!